MEET YOUR PARTNER'S SEXPECTATION:

How To Improve Your Sex Life By Satisfying Your Partner

FLORA HERRMANN

TABLE OF CONTENTS

INTRODUCTION

Role-playing games, lingerie, and romance book, according to Emily Nagoski, Ph.D., a sex educator and the author of the best-selling book "Come as You Are: The Surprising New Science That Will Transform Your Sex Life," are all fantastic methods to activate your sexual accelerator, but they typically aren't enough.

Nagoski tells NBC News BETTER, "Those things are wonderful; if you want them, go ahead. But it turns out that people are suffering generally not because there isn't enough stimulation to the accelerator — it's that there is too much stimulus to the brake."

According to Nagoski, nothing sets off your brake faster than stress: "stress is a survival strategy to aid you when your body is providing you signals that suggest you are not secure right now." If you're not safe at the time, is it OK to engage in sexual activity?

Despite your best efforts, persistent stress can entirely stifle your desire for sex, according to Nagoski. She lists a few factors that might put a brake on your progress: work, child care, and less sleep.

For couples, the pressure of maintaining a consistent sex life is a great source of stress; ironically, it is often the reason they're not having it consistently.

This book: ***MEET YOUR PARTNER'S SEXPECTATIONS*** provides couples with a thorough manual on how to get their accelerator going.

Chapter 1
FOREPLAY

Foreplay is any sexual behavior that occurs before actual sexual contact. Having said that, intercourse is optional and need not be the centerpiece of the event. When done properly, great foreplay is quite hot.

Is it important? Yes, very important? Sexual activity is made delightful and even conceivable by the physiological and physical reactions that foreplay sets off.

Physiological Reactions: Foreplay does indeed feel wonderful physically, but it also has deeper effects. By establishing emotional connection during foreplay, you and your spouse may feel closer both inside and outside of the bedroom. Not currently engaged? It's no trouble! Additionally, foreplay decreases inhibitions, which can make sex more sensual for both couples and virtual strangers.

Additionally, some foreplay could revive your libido if stress has killed it. For instance, kissing causes the release of oxytocin, dopamine, and serotonin. This chemical cocktail raises feelings of love, kinship, and happiness while decreasing cortisol (the stress hormone).

Physical Reactions: Foreplay increases sexual arousal, which should not be mistaken for sexual desire, though it can also do that. This actually gets the juices flowing. Your body's physical reactions to sexual desire include the following:

- A rise in your blood pressure, pulse, and heart rate
- Your blood vessels, especially those in your genitals, are dilated
- The labia, clitoris, and penis enlarge as a result of increased blood supply to the genital area.
- Breast swelling and erect nipples

- Lubrication of the vagina, which can improve pleasure and reduce discomfort during sexual contact

First things first: people have different interpretations of foreplay:

Foreplay is typically referred to be erotic stimulation that occurs before sexual contact. Foreplay is defined as an action or behavior that occurs before an event when sexual activity is excluded from the equation. That "event" may not appear the same to you as it does to another person, and that is totally OK.

It doesn't necessarily result in intercourse: If you don't want it to, intercourse doesn't have to be the primary "course" or even on the menu. Foreplay can actually stand on its own and be all you need to induce orgasm. It can even serve as the primary event. In reality, studies have long indicated that most females don't climax during sexual contact alone. Foreplay can thus be anything you want it to be as long as there is consent.

Even before things become heated up, you may start: You've got to start someplace, right? But who says you have to start while things are tense or even in the same room? If you know you're getting together later that day or in a few days, you can use foreplay to get the party started and keep it going. Here are some ideas to get you, well, started.

Leave a note: A note can start them off without even the requirement for creativity! It should work if you leave a letter implying that you can't wait to get dirty later on their pillow or in their workout bag.

Sext: Texting is quick, simple, and convenient. Things will definitely heat up south of the border if you send them a brief text warning them about what you're going to do to them or how hot it makes you when they [fill in the blank]. Additionally, it conveys your concern for them, and who doesn't enjoy that?

Have dinner or drinks together: Footsies below the table, a brief makeout session in the bathroom or parking lot, or a sneaky glance at what you're wearing — or not wearing — beneath your clothing. Here are a few strategies for converting a pre-fun dinner or a few drinks into foreplay.

Roleplaying: Use foreplay as a time to indulge in your most fanciful dreams. When you meet for dinner or drinks, act like you are complete strangers looking for a one-night stand. What about pretending to be a doctor and a wicked nurse? Your choice!

Give them a genuine kiss: Don't send them off or greet them with a peck; make eye contact, lean in close, and give them a passionate kiss. Make sure you moan just enough to get them excited about what's coming by using your hands and mouth.

Tell them it's Pre-game time: No need to be coy when your goal is to strip them nude and perform the unholiest of rituals. Tell them in the most vivid way possible that the one thing you want more than anything is to get them hot, hard, or wet and keep them that way all day and night. Schwing!

What if you want to initiate?

Want more than just the wham bam? With the appropriate motions, you may create the ideal atmosphere for foreplay and any other action you choose.

Light some candles: Nothing sets the mood for all the sensual things better than some lit candles. Since tea lights are cheap, stock up on them and light them in any place you could find yourself in. Did we mention that candlelight makes skin look good?

Play some music: Everybody has one or two songs that really speak to them in their own unique way. Make a playlist of others, learn what theirs is, and add yours in for good measure. Classic songs include "Let's Get it On" by Barry White and "Love to Love You" by Donna Summer. Another well-liked song is "Earned It" by The Weekend, and "Animal" by Nine Inch Nails is a hot one and my personal favorite.

Dance: Two bodies squeezed together while you sway to the beat of seductive music and feel each other's hot breath on your cheek. Enough said.

Striptease: A striptease doesn't require a pole or even very impressive motions. Dim the lights and progressively remove your garments while maintaining a fearless face. Of course, you can pretend to be very confident.

Put out an erotic spread: Prepare a variety of erotic treats for sharing and set up a picnic on the bed. Juicy strawberries and cherries are ideal for feeding — and licking off — each other, along with some whipped cream and chocolate sauce for dipping. The natural aphrodisiac is chocolate. Bon appetit!

Make out: Kick it old school. Do it against the window, on the couch, or in the back of a taxi.

Already in the moment?

It's time for outercourse (yes, that's a thing), if you're already well on your way and experiencing all the great feelings, here are some other things to try.

Massage: A sensual massage may do wonders for the body and mind, demonstrating the actual power of touch. Use massage candles, which may be extremely reminiscent of Fifty Shades of Grey, and light some candles while getting the oil ready. As you work your way up, start at their feet and be sure to touch all of their sensual pressure points while lingering where they want you to.

Erogenous zones: Your partner's body is filled with hot spots that are begging to be stroked. Work your way through all of their erogenous areas with kisses, licks, and nibbles.

Skin on skin: It turns out that dry humping isn't only for horny teenagers. It's impossible to top the exquisite anticipation of two bodies rubbing against each other in varying degrees of nakedness.

Verbalize: Talking about what you want during sexy time guarantees that you both get what you need in bed in addition to serving as foreplay. Inform them about your sexual desires and what makes you tick.

Toys: Sex toys go beyond enormous dildos in the shape of cocks. Every erogenous zone you can conceive of can be vibrated externally with vibrators of any size and form. To take foreplay to the next level, you may also utilize finger and nipple vibrations. Better information on this is provided in Chapter 6 - Toys & Lubricants.

How soapy shower: how does it feel to slide your hands around each other's body while applying hot, wet skin? Yes, please! A hot bath also works.

Sensory Play: Although all this kissing and dry humping will certainly pique the senses, you may heighten the experience with a few accessories. Tickle your companion while they are blindfolded by using objects like feathers, ice cubes, and your tongue to create varying textures and temperatures. Use items you currently own that could feel pleasant against the skin, or get an internet seduction kit.

Do you want to proceed?

Are you ready for the entree? Use these suggestions to turn it into a full-on feast of pleasure.

Oral Sex: When having oral sex, start far from the genitals and let your lips descend. The majority of the labor will be done by your lips, but don't allow your hands go inactive! While you are giving them oral gratification, use them to caress other areas of their body. Better information on this is provided in Chapter 3: Oral Sex.

Heat it up: While you're down there, don't forget to check out these less well-known but oh-so-pleasant areas: the clitoral hood, which is the flap of skin over the top of the clit, and the frenulum, which is a small skin crease on the underside of the penis where the shaft meets the head. The posture of the moment looks to be doggy! The clit, penis, perineum, and prostate are just a few of the additional areas that the penetrating partner has easy access to and may wish to love on concurrently. Reaching these may also bring about an anal orgasm in the receiving partner.

Keep it safe: Taking a hot, soapy shower together makes you completely set for anal action. Before entering all the way, it's also the ideal moment to tickle the opening with your tongue or a finger.

What if your significant other doesn't appear keen on foreplay?

Foreplay just doesn't seem to matter to certain individuals. Yes, being a lazy or selfish lover might contribute to the issue, but it could also be due to a lack of self-assurance or ignorance of the whys and hows. It can be difficult to discuss your preferences in bed, especially if you fear hurting or upsetting your partner.

Here are some ideas to ease the process:

1. Starting off on a good note: Start by telling them what they do that feels nice and how you want more of it rather than bringing up what they're not doing. For instance: "I enjoy it when you kiss my neck before our sexual encounters. I would tolerate such treatment from you all night.

2. Instead of blaming them, say that your body needs something else since it thinks they aren't pleasing it.

3. Show and tell: A person may occasionally require a little more motivation. The next time you give them a hug or kiss, linger a little longer and tell them how good it feels as you gently move their hands over your body. If their lack of interest in foreplay is due to ignorance, watching a video on tantric sex might give them a little push in the right direction.

4. Ask them what they need from you and then let them know how much you enjoy making them feel good. Inquire about any other tasks they would like you to perform. It's a fantastic way to start a conversation so that both of you can express what you want.

5. Explain to them why it matters to you: It might be necessary to be completely open and explain your need for foreplay.

Some foreplay-related points that might be worth mentioning:

- It makes you more sexually active and wetter.
- It also makes you orgasm more intensely.
- It makes you feel more connected to them since it heightens bodily awareness of pleasure zones
- Not everyone is aroused at the same rate, some require more time than others.

Conclusion:

What foreplay and sex is to you must not resemble what you see in the media. You're free to enjoy without adhering to any particular schedule or arrangement! Similar like dessert before supper, it will be delightful whenever you eat it.

Chapter 2

DIRTY TALK

To dominate the filthy talk game, you don't need to write erotica or fanfiction. You only need a little self-assurance, an open partner (or two!), and this dirty talk manual. Continue reading for a ton of instances of filthy talking you may use on your crush in any situation. Read them aloud later, copy and paste them, or just glance at them right away.

Respect and consent are essential: The author of "The Ultimate Guide to Threesomes," Stella Harris, a certified intimacy educator and sex coach, advises constantly checking in before starting any dirty chat, whether it be in person or by text.

You might say:
"I had a really erotic dream about us, and I just woke up. Can I share it with you?"

"I intend to climb into bed and indulge myself. Do you want to engage in some nasty chat while I do?"

"Do you want to hear about last night from my perspective? I can't quit thinking about it."

"If you know what I mean, I'm in a mood. Would you be interested in exchanging some explicit texts?"

"During sex, I occasionally speak rather filthily. I just want to gauge your reaction before we move on. Do you love using foul language during sex?"

It's also a good idea to share any no-fly trigger phrases at the beginning of a conversation. To ensure that the filthy discussion is within everyone's predetermined bounds and preferences, discuss what it will involve, according to Harris.

For instance, although "soft" may be a complement to you, your spouse may see it as a critique of their weight. Or perhaps you enjoy being referred to as a "slut" while having sex, but asking your partner to do so makes them uncomfortable. Like you would with any other sex, she explains, you should bargain dirty talk in advance.

Here's how that may appear:

"Just so you know, I truly enjoy the adjectives 'strong' and 'competent' being used to describe me in bed and detest any phrases that would indicate I'm not all muscle. Do you wish to share any adjective preferences with me?"

"Are there any nicknames you enjoy hearing in bed? 'Baby'? 'Slut'? "Dad's girl" "My young girl?"

"Before we get started, I just want to let you know that I find allusions to doggy style to be triggering. Therefore, I'd prefer to avoid including that in our verbal and physical play. Do you have a preferred method?"

"I prefer having my chest called my 'chest' and my genitals called my 'click' or 'cock. Are there any terms you favor or dislike for the sections of your body?"

Everyone gets apprehensive when it comes to sex, at least occasionally, according to Harris. "Confidence is vital, even if it might feel tough to pull off at first." You should read Thomas Nielson's book HOW TO BE CONFIDENT, which is the definitive manual on how to develop confidence. Fake it till you make it if you don't already have it. This is how:

No matter how you're feeling in general, lead with excitement. People might feel liked and desired if you show passion for what you're doing and the person you're with, according to Harris. What if they feel wanted? They'll have a better chance of making you experience the same emotion. In addition, she adds, "it'll probably make the person you're with courageous and say or do new things too." Win-win!

Try not to overthink it. Can you imagine a complex fantasy involving handcuffs, a dragon that breathes fire, and a multi-orgasmic sex session? Yes, provided your partner and you both agree to engage in that particular type of linguistic hanky-panky. Simply state what you're doing or what you'd want to be doing! Harris advises students to "describe everything using all five senses." What can you feel, hear, see, and smell right now? Describe that!

Make sounds: whether you're speaking or sharing audio notes with someone. You can urge your companion to continue talking or acting by saying "mmm," "oh baby," or other sounds that are reminiscent of moans.

Ask your spouse a question: If you run into trouble, here is another alternative.
For instance, "Hmm, and what do you want me to do for you?"
"Is that what you want? Please elaborate"
"Yeah? What would you do next?"
"And what follows?"
When you text instead of speaking in person, you have the gift of time. It's time to express your experience fully and to think of new ways to say things.

Building Anticipation:
"When I get home, I can't wait to send you a picture of my new underwear"
"Baby, I'm going to make you orgasm with just my words when I get home from work."
"Will you behave well tonight for Mommy?"

At the time:
"I feel very seductive. Do you have the okay to touch me, Master?
"I wish you could feel what you do to my body by reaching between my legs."
"When I shut my eyes, I almost physically see how your hands follow the contours of my body and how your fingertips pinpoint the locations of my hot points"

Requests
"Exactly describe to me your memory of our first sex session."
"Go into more detail for me. Don't leave anything out at all"

"If I came to your door wearing my uniform, what would you do to me, please?"

Recognitions:
"You always know what to say"
"You're able to make my pulse race, my eyes roll back, and my breath catch with a single text."
"E.L. James, are you there? Kidding. However, those are some hot messages you came up with tonight, dammit"

Afterward:
"I can't wait to see what you can do to my body with your tongue and hands—if you're interested, that is—after witnessing what you can do to it with only words, of course."
"Wow. I was shocked at how sexy that was! If you liked that, too, I'd love to do that again someday"
"I'm worn out from that orgasm. But first, I want to ask: Is there anything I can do for you to be satisfied with how this conversation concluded before I put my phone down"

If you enjoy leaving voicemails or using the phone

Using your voice to improve your sexting session? Use these one-liners to sound like a nasty talking professional or a phone sex operator! Have faith—your boo won't realize what struck them.

Building anticipation:

"I'm going to pull my jeans off so I can think about you while I can touch myself more readily"

"I'm so excited to make you curse my name tonight"

"I'm going to contact you when you finish working and take you out for several orgasms"

At the time:

"Consider this: You're reading on your bed. I exit the restroom wearing silk. My lips are already opened, eager to receive you into my mouth, and my breasts are oozing out of the fabric. My legs are tanned from the summer.

"I'm thinking back to when you gave me a taste in the fields. The way you snuck your head beneath my summer dress, crept between my legs, and licked me like a dog licks its dish. Up until I dragged you on top of me, you kept tasting things with your fingers and tongue in alternation"
"On CrashPad, I viewed a pornographic film. Can I share it with you?"

Requests:
"Please remove your underwear for me, please. Will you comply?"
"Send me the URL of your favorite pornographic video. As I f*ck my little, cramped hole, I want to see it and think about you"

Recognitions:
"I adore how your voice sounds when you're bursting with want."
"You say the dirtiest things for a decent boy. I also adore it.

"When I say anything that makes you feel attracted to me, I love to hear your breath catch in your throat"

Afterward:
"Wow, I didn't know phone sex could be so enjoyable. I appreciate you letting me be a part of that event. The next time you want to do that, give me a call"
"Honey, that was hot, damn. How did it make you feel?"
"Would you mind talking to me on the phone while I simply breathe to get over that orgasm?"

When you video chat. Setting the environment is the first step in effective video sex, according to Harris. Spend some time considering your surroundings. What about the lighting? How do your angles look so far? Candles should be lit, she advises. This will put you and your companions in the right frame of mind.

Use these lines to start after you've completed that:

Building Anticipation:
"I want you to push yourself harder than you did the last time we played tonight on video"
"I'm going to fill my gorgeous bussy with the dildo you gave me for my birthday later tonight. If you agree to make it worthwhile for me, I'll let you watch"
"Today, I'm sporting the boxers you adore. At 8:00 p.m., if you're available, you may see me take them off"

At the time:
"If I was with you I'd lay you across my lap and take my time with that perfect ass. I would start by drawing small, delicate circles over each cheek while gradually bringing my fingertips closer to your ideal hole. I would then make you beg for me to touch you as you were writhing over my lap. I would only approach the nerve-wracking entrance when you said "please" and drive you crazy"

"Go ahead, use the toy I normally use to play with you. Use it on yourself the same way I would on you by starting at your nipples and working your way down to your lips, labia, and then your exquisite little bud"
"I can feel the heat of your body on mine when I close my eyes. when you push against my body, how it comes from your body"

Requests:
"I adore it when we delve deeper into kinky dreams. Can we, however, keep it a bit more subdued tonight?"
"Tell me about your most recent threesome. Don't leave anything out."
"I want to impersonate holding your hands. Please specify how I should touch myself"

Recognitions:
"I don't think anyone has ever made me this hot without really touching me before."
"Wow… I didn't believe I could ever desire you more. After that, though, I do"
"You are just very seductive"

Afterward:

"I need to end the conversation since I have a client call in 30 minutes. But I would want to do this again tomorrow. Say, 7 p.m.?"

"Oof! After that, I need water and a burger! In the best manner conceivable, I'm exhausted. Is there anything I can Uber Eats to you?"

"I am aware that you enjoy snuggling after having sex. Is there anything I can do today to give us that same experience?"

If you're in person: Whether you can be "physically intimate" at that particular time will determine what you say.

You two are out in public together:

"If these people weren't present, I would fall to my knees"

"I keep picturing me dragging you into the coat closet, stuffing my underwear down your throat, and f*cking your ravenous hole"

"I want you to recall the sensation I had inside you the previous evening without letting desire color your features. I was drawn deeper by the way your body surged around me, gripped onto me"

"I'll help you come over and over when we go back to the hotel room"

You're in a private area:
"While I taste you, tell me about the porn you saw last night."

"Tonight , honey, I'm going to tease the living crap out of you"

"My favorite flavor is you. I could spend the entire night between your legs"

"You look so sexy as you lay there waiting for my ravishment"

If you want more motivation
Harris suggests reading erotica, seeing some R-rated movies, or listening to some "suggestive" podcasts for even more inspiration. When the inspiration comes from an outside source, she explains, "it might be simpler to start."

No big deal if you feel like you "messed up" or just aren't feeling it. Just communicate exactly what happened or what you're feeling and ask for what you want (or need) to happen next.

If your tongue became stuck
"My apologies! I have no idea why I said it. I felt anxious. Let me try again?"
"Oh my goodness, I'm so excited that I can't speak"
"I have no idea what to say because I'm so hot"
"I'm sorry; I should have asked your permission before calling you that. I should have done that without a doubt. I apologize. What do you think about being called that during sex, please? I could call you about so many other things instead!"
"WOW! I should have checked the temperature there before I went. I'm sorry; I was just caught up in the moment"

If you decide to stop or try another option
"I know I mentioned earlier today that I was really looking forward to experiencing phone

sex, but now that we're really doing it, my fears are getting the better of me. Can we pause for now and attempt over text again later today or tomorrow?"

"Last time we had sex was amazing, but I was wondering if tonight we might try exchanging audio notes?"

"I'll be honest: I'm having difficulties getting out of work mode this evening. Can we simply speak about our days and put the hot stuff on hold?"

"I am aware that you didn't mean for this to happen, but what you just said set off a trauma reaction to something that occurred a few years ago. I'll thus put a stop to this discussion and take care of myself. However, I'd love to give this another go in a few days. Let me text you."

Congrats! you've made it to the conclusion of this nasty talk class and passed with flying colors.

Chapter 3

ORAL SEX

First things first: don't worry if this is your first dive; everyone has to start somewhere. However, we want to be sure that everything is okay because life is too short to waste on some mediocre orals. After all, if you're gonna go down, you should do it well. Here is all you need to know about having and receiving oral sex, as well as all the amusing and sometimes useful information in between.

Let's clarify the situation.
Let's speak about the gritty first before getting down to nitty.

Oral sex is "real" sex, yes.
Ignore whatever Clinton or anyone else has told you about what sex is and isn't. The only kind of sex is not penis-in-vagina intercourse. In certain cases, oral sex might even be more enjoyable than penetrative sex.

Try not to spend too much time worrying about how your vulva and penises compare to those of other people because your body is unique. Penises aren't often large or smooth like an eggplant emoji, and vulvas don't always resemble a fully ripe peach.

Everyone has some sort of scent; you can scrub all you want, but it will still be there. It's okay to have what is known as your natural odor. Nevertheless, freshening up before having oral sex is merely polite.

To Keep Things Fresh:
- Take a bath or shower, or at the very least wash your genital area with soap and water.
- In the event that you suddenly need to freshen up, use a moist paper towel or unscented wipes.
- Deodorants and fragrances shouldn't be used there since they aren't healthy for the genitals.

Everyone also has a taste: Whose genital juice has a cookies-and-cream flavor, do you know? No one has! We all have a taste down there. You should taste okay as long as you're in good health and practice good cleanliness. If you're still concerned about becoming funky spunk, changing your diet may make your juice taste better. Garlic, onions, asparagus, and cabbage should be avoided since they purportedly have an unappealing flavor. Try eating pineapple, papaya, nutmeg, cinnamon, and celery to sweeten your sauce.

Common Questions Men Ask:

1. "Do you truly flick the clit?" You may! It might be enjoyable to gently flick the clit with your tongue to change things up and increase enjoyment. Instead of a woodpecker decimating a tree, picture a gentle puppy tongue licking an ice cream cone.

2. Should you stick to non-penetration or insert your tongue? That depends on the

person you're going down with. Some individuals find the mere thought of having their tongues poked scorching AF, but less feeling results from fewer nerve endings in the opening. Go to town if they enjoy it.

3. What if they are either pregnant or on their period? Go forward if they agree and you are comfortable with it. Focusing on the clit is definitely the best course of action because things may become nasty. Be aware that blood might taste metallic and have an odor. If you're uncomfortable, a dental dam can assist.

Technique: Try These Postures:
Long strokes over their underwear with your tongue flat will make the material wet - and them too.
Spend some time licking the flesh mound above the clit before putting your tongue to their skin. Give their inner thighs some attention as well.

Then, lick your way up, laying your moist tongue flat at the base of their vulva. Repeat.

The clitoral hood, the little flap of skin above the clit, may be licked in tiny circles by flexing your tongue and using the tip.

To direct your tongue's tip toward the clit, softly lift the hood up with your fingers. Increase pressure and speed gradually after a mild start.

Keep going until you find a rhythm that they enjoy to push them over the brink.

Positions:

Almost any penetrative sex position may be converted to an oral sex position with a little effort and creativity. But we advise adopting the following postures to prevent neck pain:

- Lie Back and Enjoy: Have them lie on their backs with their legs spread and a cushion under their butt, and then lie back and take it all in as you kneel or squat between them with your face in the muck.
- Control Freak: Lie on your back with them straddling your face while they are

facing you, allowing them to control the pressure and movements, and watch you work for it.

- Almost 69: They get to straddle your face once more, but this time they're facing your main draw and can repay the favor with some 69 action.

Safety and cleanup are both taken care of by a quick wash with soap and water or soft wipes before and after oral sex.

Common Questions Women Ask:

1. what do I do if he is not circumcised? Regarding the technique between circumcised and uncircumcised people, there are little differences. Let the foreskin go up and down with your hand if you start with a hand job. Pull the foreskin gently down to reveal the head when you're ready to get licky with it.

2. Have you got a deep throat? Not unless you want to, of course. An oral session

won't be made or broken by not digging deep enough. By resting the tip of your tongue on the roof of your mouth and sucking as much as you like without an abrupt gag, you can completely imitate it.

3. Should you swallow ejaculate, spit it out, or keep it out of your mouth entirely? You should first discuss that with your spouse, but you are never required to do something you don't want to do. Having them finish on your chin, closed lips, or any other location you feel comfortable with should work if it's a visual turn on for your partner.

Technique: Try These Postures:
Start by tracing the base of their shaft with the tip of your tongue, pausing to go around their head.

Give the shaft's underside some tender loving care, and then with the tip of your tongue, gently wiggle the frenulum, the little fold of skin where the shaft meets the head.

Lap up the entire length and repeat: If you tell them how much you like doing it, bonus points. When you move up and down while gently sucking, hold the base of their shaft in your hand and take the remainder of it in your mouth. accelerate as their pleasure increases.

Positions:

Once more, use your imagination to find a position where you can get a good blow. Try the following:

- Open Wide: While they stand with their head facing your feet and penis covering your mouth, lie on your bed with your head close to the edge.
- Sit and Suck: Two ways to use one chair. You may either do the sitting while they stand with their legs on each side of the chair as you lean in and take matters into your mouth, or you can have them sit on the chair.
- Laidback Lovin':This BJ position is by far the most comfortable one ever, and it's

ideal for those leisurely morning blow jobs. Use their body as a pillow when they are on their back while you are lying on your side and using your lips and hands.

Flavored condoms are our solution for both safety and cleanliness. Seriously, flavored condoms lower your risk for STIs while offering you something sweet to suck on if you want to perform a safe blowout. Cleaning up is as simple as taking a shower before and after.

Common Questions on Giving a Rim Work:
1. Are you going to get poop in your mouth? It's a possibility, I won't lie. The residues of feces that persist in the anus may typically be removed by washing with a soft cloth, soap, and water.

2. What do you do if there's hair back there: No huge deal. Unless they want their bottom shaved, just go along with it; however, that is a whole other subject.

3. Should you stick to non-penetration or stick your tongue out? Your degree of comfort is everything. There is no excuse for sticking your tongue out in inappropriate places. Fingers and butt plugs can perform the penetration for you if they're receptive to it.

Technique: Try these beginning to end motions:

Start by briefly kissing and licking their cheeks.

Just below the hole, place your tongue flat and at ease. Then, slowly lick up and down.

Use your tongue's tip to run circles around the hole, beginning with light pressure and increasing it as their level of enjoyment increases.

If both of you have consented to penetration, go ahead and softly press a tongue, finger, or sex object into the anus.

Once they're happy, keep using your tongue on, between, or around the perineum.

Position:

Doggy style is a favorite position for rimming. You have equal control over the pressure and movement to choose what is most comfortable for you both. They should get down on all fours as you take a knee behind. They can put a pillow under their head and raise or tuck their bottom up to your lips.

Safety and cleanup: For safe rimming, either a dental dam, a tongue condom, or a standard condom used as a dam will work. If you're going to use your fingers in or near the anus, it's also crucial to have clean hands and well-trimmed nails. The receiver can choose to use an enema, but a thorough washing of the region in the bath or shower with mild soap and water is adequate. After finishing, you have the option of using an oral rinse or brushing your teeth. Perhaps you should wash your face and hands as well.

General Tips: Now that you know the motions, here are some general pointers. Make oral sex the pleasureable by using these suggestions:

Ask your companion: Making any sort of sex as good as it can be requires asking questions. Be careful to gain their unambiguous permission before proceeding. Not only is it a good idea to find out what makes people tick, but doing so may be foreplay. Asking questions when giving an oral is nice, so don't be shy about doing so.

Use your breath to explain why it would feel amazing on their skin: It's hot and somewhat humid. Let your hot breath linger just an inch over their skin while you tease them into a frenzy.

Make some sounds and let them know how much you are enjoying yourself. It's okay to groan, sputter, and slurp!

Lock eyes: Making eye contact while you go down is hot AF. Additionally, it's a terrific method to see how your spouse responds to your activities so you can see what works and what doesn't.

Work with your hands: Don't be afraid to use them! Use them to widen the labia for easier access to all the crevices or to manipulate the shaft expertly while circling their head with your tongue.

Look beyond these areas: To increase the orgasmic intensity of oral play, explore their other erogenous zones with your lips, hands, or sex toys.

Put some lubricant in the mix Sure, your tongue is very juicy, but lubricating is enjoyable for everyone! Flavored lubes can improve hand activity or toy play as well as oral sex.

Take it to the edge: The ultimate orgasm-inducing tease is edging, often known as orgasm control. You use your powers to push them just over the point of climax, then you pause for approximately 30 seconds before resuming the stimulation.

Conclusion:

If you really get into it, oral sex can be as enjoyable for the giver as it is for the recipient. To put it another way, leave your inhibitions outside and don't be scared to get dirty. Bon appetit!

Chapter 4

SEX POSITIONS

The Kama Sutra, an old Indian book on sexuality, demonstrates that sexual activity is an endless pursuit of variety. There are countless hot sex positions for couples that combine the bodies of men and women for their enjoyment. Knowing different sex positions can make you a better and more creative lover for your partner if you're in a heterosexual relationship.

How Can You Have Sex That Is Mutually Satisfying?

Every couple will receive a different response. "According to Tameca Harris-Jackson, PhD, LCSW, a certified sex educator and sex therapist and the founder of Hope and Serenity Health Services, a counseling facility in Altamont Springs, Florida, the best position is the one that benefits the individual or individuals involved. "According to Harris-Jackson, experimenting with various sex positions actually presents a chance to introduce various ways of experiencing pleasure into sexual intimacy and a sexual relationship. "Eating the same thing every day for 20 years doesn't guarantee that you'll enjoy it the most. Simply put, you are receiving nutrients. However, if you try to add some parsley to that meal, you might taste it differently and it might turn into a more interesting meal. And that's what changing roles can do to a relationship.

There are other nonphysical aspects to take into account. Consider intimacy as an example. Intimacy may result in greater sexual experiences for many individuals, especially women, since partners feel safe and trustworthy enough to express their desires and attempt new things.

According to studies supported by the Kinsey Institute at the University of Indiana that looked at sex during the early stages of the COVID-19 epidemic in 2020, many couples are discovering precisely those advantages. In spite of having less frequent sex in the early weeks of the epidemic, individuals were more open to trying new things, including as sexting, exchanging sexual fantasies, and trying out novel sex positions, according to a poll of 1,559 adults conducted online. The journal Leisure Sciences published a commentary on the findings in its June 2020 edition.

Why It's Important to Try New Sexual Positions:

According to study coauthor Justin L. Lehmiller, PhD, research fellow at the Kinsey Institute in Bloomington, Indiana, and host of the Sex and Psychology Podcast, "We know that this has been a really stressful period of time and that can make it hard to get aroused and stay aroused." "Trying new things can increase your level of arousal. Discovering what works for your body and your relationship via trying new things will have long-term rewards. These maneuvers can be effective even if you are not an expert gymnast. To increase the heat between the sheets, avoid thinking about "crazy sex positions" and instead consider novel sex positions.

Dr. Lehmiller affirms that "not every position is for everyone and that's alright." But it doesn't mean you shouldn't attempt new and different things even if the postures discussed here don't work for you (or if you've already tried them). One of the things that keeps us interested in returning for more is novelty. We tend to lose interest in sex when it occurs frequently. A convenient method to inject some variety and newness into our sexual life is by taking on new positions.

1. The Missionary Position or Face to Face: It's a straightforward sex position: The woman is spread-eagled on her back, her knees slightly bowed. While supporting his body weight with his arms or elbows, the male slides his penis inside her vagina while lying between her legs.

The issue with this sexual position is that it doesn't give ladies as much pleasure as other positions do. In this posture, the man's pelvis can occasionally stimulate the clitoris and provides incredible closeness through face-to-face contact. However, the penis's orientation prevents deep penetration or G-spot activation (felt through a location on the front wall of the vagina, and believed by some experts to be a stimulus for orgasm in women). Some women also claim that the clitoral stimulation in this sex position is insufficient to induce climax.

2. Woman on Top or a Cowgirl: The lady kneels in front of the guy while straddling his pelvis and guiding his penis into her vagina in this sex position. The male is lying on his back. She can then lie on him or stand up. According to Dr. Harris-Jackson, "this is a fantastic position for a woman to regulate the degree of penetration." She has complete control over how much penis she wants when she's on top. "It's also a good place to get a variety of stimuli. The woman's nipples might be engaged while her torso is upright, which can cause an increase in arousal. Having access to the clitoris for stimulation is advantageous.

Additionally, the lady has the option to bounce up and down, grind, or create hip circles, each of which produces a little different experience. If a person has back problems, Harris-Jackson adds, "this is also a nice posture for them since it's virtually a resting position." Men who are highly sensitive to visual cues can recline and observe their female companion.

3. Reverse Rider on Top or Reverse Cowgirl: The lady sits astride him, facing her partner's feet, and puts the penis into her vagina as the guy rests on his back on the bed. The woman has control over the thrusts' tempo and rhythm. For the penetrating partner, who gets to watch his partner's back and buttocks, this position can be especially exciting. The experience can be improved for both parties by pinching or grabbing the buttocks. Since the woman must either lean back or sit up straight to fit the penis' angle, this posture can be challenging to learn.

According to Harris-Jackson, having your partner bend his knees and then bracing yourself with your hands against his thighs, placing your hands behind you on his waist, or placing your hands on pillows on either side of him can prevent the man from feeling pain and discomfort because it may feel as though his penis is breaking.

Switch it Up: According to Lorrae Jo Bradbury, sex and love coach and creator of SluttyGirlProblems.com and LorraeJo.com, "This may be one of those positions that is better in principle than in practice." Consider using it as a pre-intercourse foreplay position by grinding on his penis.

4. Rear entry or doggy style: The woman is in this position, kneeling on her hands and knees, supporting herself. From behind, he penetrates her vagina while squatting. The finest sex position for deep vaginal penetration is this one. The guy is free to push his pelvis quickly and forcefully, and he may caress a large portion of the woman's body. Additionally, the posture enables effective G-spot stimulation.

Switch It Up: Because there is no face-to-face contact, some women say that this sex position is too impersonal. Moving your legs closer to your chest and arching your back will allow your partner to lean into you close to your face, allowing you to create closer eye contact, advises Bradbury. You can also try this posture in front of a mirror so you can see each other's faces, advises Bradbury.

The study, which was published in the August 2020 issue of Sexual Medicine, examined 13 various sex positions and discovered that the doggy position is not often linked to female orgasms. Continue exploring if it doesn't work for you or your spouse.

5. The Corkscrew: As her partner enters her vagina from behind, the lady leans forward on the edge of the bed, resting on her hip and forearm. For a firmer grip on the penis, the woman can keep her thighs close together. However, if she spreads her legs, the clitoris is visible and may be stroked as a guy pushes her from behind. Although this position may be simpler and more comfortable, Bradbury claims "You're getting that deeper penetration like doggy style, but this may be an easier and more comfortable position".

Switch It Up: According to Bradbury, the clitoris is within easy reach and your partner can easily lean down to make out with you.

6. **Side by Side or Sideways:** The couple is lying side by side, facing each other. In order for the man to insert his penis, the woman lifts her top leg. The leg can then be used to cross his leg or wrap around his waist. According to Bradbury, this position is ideal for morning sex when you might be a little sleepy. As a result of your proximity to your partner's face, it provides a great deal of closeness. During the act of making love, the lovers may kiss and caress one another. The sex position is comfortable, doesn't

demand much energy from either party, and provides a chance for effective clitoral stimulation.

Swutch It Up: According to Bradbury, penetration can be increased if the lady drapes both of her legs over her partner's waist. This gives the clitoris easy access and makes it possible to stimulate it with a finger or a toy. "Everyone should be in this position, in my opinion. Additionally, it provides cuddling comfort.

7. Lazy Dog or Flat Iron: The woman is positioned on the bed face down, her legs straight and her hips slightly raised. Put a cushion beneath your hips (if you choose). From behind, her partner penetrates her vagina. The woman's legs will be closer together while she is on her stomach, which will result in a tighter fit for her partner's penis. This can result in a brand-new, stronger feeling. According to Harris-Jackson, "this is a really wonderful method to intensify the sense of tightness for the penetrating partner." Because the partner can reach around with his hand or a sex toy to provide dual stimulation, it's also beneficial for clitoral stimulation. Additionally, you're positioning your body in such a way that the penis is perfectly aligned to stroke against the G-spot, making it an ideal posture for G-spot stimulation.

8. Face-Off: This might be a more effective missionary position as there is considerable eye contact and clitoral stimulation. In this position, the woman climbs onto the man's lap and wraps her legs behind him while he sits on the edge of the bed or in a comfortable seated position. The lady has control over how quickly she thrusts. Direct clitoral stimulation and eye contact are also possible in this posture, which can improve intimacy.

Bonus: You can touch and caress your partner's body almost anywhere you choose because your hands are free. According to Harris-Jackson, "this is a particularly effective position for persons who get aroused with eye contact." "It's like missionary, only you're actually face to face. The fenale is also relieved of some of the work since her partner can raise and lower her by putting his hands on her hips.

Switch It Up: The Lotus position is extremely similar to the face-off position, with the exception that the male sits cross-legged on a bed or chair.

9. Pretzel Dip: The man is straddling the right leg of the woman, who is lying on her right side. The male then enters the vagina while pulling his partner's left leg up and around his left side. In addition to providing for close eye contact, this posture enables for thorough penetration.

Switch it Up: According to Bradbury, "you may also take your left leg and draw it toward your chest to obtain a deeper angle." And both spouses have incredible access to the clitoris. You'll have free hands, so you may examine each other's bodies thoroughly. Harris-Jackson adds: Depending on your angle, this posture may also provide G-spot stimulation.

10. The Coital Alignment Technique, or CAT: Roll with CAT if you prefer to rock rather than thrust. The key distinction between this position and the missionary is that in this one, the guy pushes his base of the penis until it aligns with the clitoris and the two body parts come into touch. Once they do, they continue to rock back and forth while staying in close proximity. Lehmiller describes it as "a somewhat different style of having sex." You sway back and forth as opposed to thrusting. Because she is constantly stimulated, doing so lengthens the duration of the encounter for the guy and enhances the likelihood that a woman will experience an orgasm.

Keep Switching It Up: Sexual Variety Is Everything!
According to Harris-Jackson, we have a strong tendency to be goal-oriented in our daily lives. "When we wake up in the morning, we have to

rush to leave the house, have our breakfast, and get to work. In both our bodies and minds, it causes a great deal of stress and tension. Many of the patients I see feel that having sex has become just one more thing they need to go and do. However, sexual partners should truly enjoy each other's company. It might be quite beneficial to change postures to reignite the connection. So, trying something new may be advantageous and enjoyable.

Chapter 5

ORGASMS

Do your orgasms fizzle more often than they sizzle? Here's a guide on how to advance sexually. If your climaxes feel like a lot of labor for little reward, there may be a medical or psychological explanation for this, a technical issue, or you may just need some assistance from some "friends." Keep trying; assistance is on the way. "It is a gift to be able to experience a strong, pleasurable orgasm. Can anything be done when our libido is down, we can't orgasm, or the quality of our orgasm isn't as powerful as it once was? Plenty!" exclaims Evelyn Hecht, CEO of New York City's EMH Physical Therapy.

Put your mind on the task. "Focus, Focus, Focus" Ellen Barnard, a sex educator, sex counselor, and spokesman for the American Association of Sexuality Educators, Counselors, and Therapists, asserts that you must be totally present. Put your cell phone somewhere you won't see it and turn it off. Stop using email. Lock the door or at least send the kids to Grandma's. When you are preoccupied with life, you are effectively watching sex from the stands when you need to be paying attention to the game. "Pay attention to how your body feels, to your knowledge of pleasure, and to the sensations themselves. Simply bring your focus back when it starts to stray to your to-do list, advises Barnard.

According to a research that appeared in the Journal of Sexual Research's September 2017 edition, either a four- or an eight-session mindfulness program for women boosted orgasm capacity by 30%. (1)

Unknown Sexual Pleasure Zones: Investigate Locations Other Than the Typical Hot Spots; Keep in mind that your body contains several nerve endings; you are more than simply your genitals. The sensation and orgasmic potential might be enhanced by tapping into your untapped (everyone has distinct unknown sexual pleasure zones). According to Michael Krychman, MD, executive director of the Southern California Center for Sexual Health in Newport Beach, California, body mapping is a fantastic technique to do this. Each couple first sketches the front and back of their bodies, after which they add lines where they want to be touched, are open to trying something new, and where they want to avoid being touched. You may utilize color coding: green indicates moving forward quickly, red indicates avoiding the area, and yellow indicates moving forward slowly and obeying directions. Then each party clarifies their meanings to the other. "This improves sexual communication and increases the likelihood that you'll experience the right level of excitement. You may avoid getting into a rut and leave room for changes in your body, appetite, and way of life if you periodically update the map, says Dr. Krychman.

Vaginal Versus Clitoral Orgasms: Not either-or. Let's also dispel the fallacy that all women can come by vaginal stimulation alone. According to a study appearing in the Journal of Sex and Marital Therapy on February 17, 2018, "while 18.4% of women reported that intercourse alone was sufficient for orgasm, 36.6% reported clitoral stimulation was necessary for orgasm during intercourse, and an additional 36% indicated that, while clitoral stimulation was not needed, their orgasms feel better if their clitoris is stimulated during intercourse."

Seek Medical Attention from Your Doctor: The capacity to experience orgasm can be impacted by a number of conditions (diabetes, selective serotonin reuptake inhibitors, anticonvulsants), as well as drugs. For problems like trouble becoming aroused, trouble attaining or keeping an erection, and a general lack of feeling during arousal or orgasm, according to Barnard, you should seek medical help.

What Condition Is Your Pelvic Floor In? Did you know that there are professionals that specialize in pelvic therapy? If you believe that physical therapy may be required, you can get your condition evaluated by these professionals. "Your pelvic floor muscles need to be relaxed throughout the day, not in a high tension condition, always on alert, to have a truly excellent orgasm. Most individuals are unaware that their pelvic floor is tensed up like a fist, which can cause painful sex with women, trouble getting and keeping an erection in men, and the capacity to climax in both cases, according to Hecht.

Pelvic muscles and What's Necessary for Effective Orgasmic Contractions: Some physical therapy centers, like the Herman and Wallace Pelvic Rehabilitation Institute, focus on pelvic floor health in addition to more visible exercises like Pilates or yoga, which help strengthen the pelvic floor while working out your entire body. In order to get a proper orgasmic contraction, the pelvic muscles must go from a totally relaxed long state to a fully tight short state; otherwise, you won't experience the whole Monty. Exercises to relax certain muscles should be done.

Hecht advises the following exercises to loosen up stiff pelvic muscles:

- Happy baby pose: Bring both knees up to your chest while lying on your back. Straighten your lower legs out in front of you while bending at the knees. Hold on by the soles and keep your feet flexed. Your knees should be drawn toward the floor as you pull your feet back. Your pelvic floor is being stretched and made more pliable.

- Inner Thigh Groin Stretch: sit on the floor with your legs as far out to the sides as possible. Lean forward and then over each leg, breathing rhythmically as you do so to feel a stretch in your inner thighs.

- Kegels done correctly starts by tightening your anal and vaginal region for five seconds. Take a breath through it. Avoid contracting your abdominal or butt muscles. up to 10 seconds of work. Release gradually and unwind completely. Prior to attempting once more, wait 10 seconds. Work up to 10 seconds, then take a 20-second break. 10 times through. then squeeze more quickly: Give the anal-vaginal region a quick squeeze before relaxing for two seconds. Inhale during the relaxation while exhaling in time with the squeeze. Perform two sets of 10 repetitions every day. Kegel exercises bolster and steady the core.

Toys Aren't Just for Kids: Fill Your Sexual Toy Chest!

There are several devices on the market designed to boost stimulation or your capacity to sense feeling in various places of your body. Nipple stimulation may occur along with other forms of stimulation. Since everyone is unique, find out what works for you. You don't need need a partner for this, so go ahead!

This brings us to the next chapter…

Chapter 6

TOYS & LUBRICANTS

Can Sex Toys Improve Your Sex Life?
Yes!

The usage of sex toys by couples might enhance their sexual connection while being frequently perceived as a lonely pastime. A great approach to spice up your relationship and increase closeness is by using a sex toy. Using a sex toy has several advantages, including helping to keep your libido stimulated and your Kegel muscles toned.

What justifies my usage of a sex toy?
The advantages of utilizing a sex toy are substantial. By elevating your mood and making you feel wonderful physically, having amazing sex may boost health and well-being. Utilizing a sex toy may liven up a stale sexual relationship and add a little pleasure to your life. The release of "feel good elements" during an orgasm is

aided by the use of a sex toy, which also improves circulation. Additionally, it can improve the flexibility and tone of the vaginal walls and encourage the discharge of vaginal secretions, which might lessen with age, due to illness, or as a side effect of medicine.

Male sex toys provide various sexual stimulation that is not possible during penetrative sex, which can aid to enhance or raise erectile function.

Sexual intercourse is simply one method to have meaningful sex; sex is more than just that. In the event when penetration is not feasible, using a sex toy may be really enjoyable for both of you. Using a sex toy may be helpful since many couples struggle to have sex because of mental or emotional issues.

Glass and metal sex toys are excellent for temperature play since they can be gradually warmed in warm water or chilled in the refrigerator (not the freezer or boiling water) for a very distinct kind of sexual experience that many people adore.

Will it sabotage my regular sex life?
Sex toys provide couples the chance to completely express their sexuality and heighten their sexual enjoyment when utilized with their partners, especially when used to excite their partners.

Sex toys may be used by couples to increase their level of sexual satisfaction, provide diversity to a potentially monotonous relationship, and make sex enjoyable. A sex toy may make sexual activity more enjoyable, interesting, and exciting. Having sex with the same person for a long time might get a little boring.

They are also an excellent method to learn new techniques that could lead to orgasm, especially if you have trouble doing thatt during penetrative sex.

Using a sex toy to get excited is no different from being excited in any other manner, and it could even make you happier. In order to avoid an aching hand if it takes a while, especially as you age, your spouse might choose to stimulate you using a sex toy.

I wish I could, but I'm too ashamed:
Since the infamous rabbit vibrator was featured on "Sex and the City," owning sex toys is now considered respectable. Recent data shows that 75% of women who possess sex toys are married and that around 60% of women own sex toys. You might be shocked to learn that most of your quieter friends have toys. A man may also have pleasure with his sex toys.

My spouse doesn't like the notion:
If your partner doesn't like the thought of you using a sex toy, do it alone or attempt to convince them that it doesn't replace them but rather enhances what you currently share. It could strengthen your relationship with your lover and foster more trust. There's a chance

you'll discover your inner sex kitten, which many partners will like.

I don't want to terrify my partner:
Some guys fear that a vibrator could replace them since they can't compete with what a sex toy can achieve. This is completely incorrect. In order to enhance their sex life, one-third of Brits admitted to using sex toys. When two people use sex toys together, their sexual pleasure is increased.

You don't have to get the largest vibrator that is offered. Bigger isn't always better; what counts is the vibrational power and where and how you want to employ it. Additionally, you don't want to scare off your companion. Many people who have never used a vibrator before start out with a smaller toy and move to a larger one as needed.

To increase your enjoyment, I advise using a pH-balanced sexual lubricant that is skin-safe. While silicone lubricants are good for use with glass, metal, or ABS plastic, they are not advised for use with silicone sex toys.

No one sex toy is suitable for everyone. Finding the ideal toys for you will need some experimentation with a range of brands because everyone's sexual requirements are different. Both sexes can enjoy a variety of sex toys that are readily available. Don't give up if you have a terrible experience with one toy; try another. Don't be scared to use a sex toy since you could discover that after you've convinced your partner to try one, they'll be addicted and want to try more.

I don't feel comfortable getting one from a store: Purchasing sex toys has never been simpler thanks to the internet. Make sure the store you choose has an email address, a phone number, and a contact address listed on their website.

A lot of phony and used sex toys that are sold online are damaging to your sexual health and enjoyment, so be aware of really inexpensive goods. It's crucial to check that a product is skin safe before purchasing it if it will come into contact with your genitals. Rubber and jelly are porous materials that are difficult to clean and can be dangerous. This indicates that germs may remain on the item and cause you to develop thrush. They also include phthalates, a chemical that is prohibited in children's toys because it poses a health risk. I suggest selecting skin-safe sex toys to safeguard your sexual well-being and enjoyment. All sex toys—silicone, metal, and glass—are safe to use and simple to clean because to their non-porous nature.

You must ensure that your information is not shared with outside parties in order to avoid receiving a barrage of unsolicited emails or catalogs. A credible business wouldn't act in this manner. If you are not tech savvy, you may also discover advertisements for luxury sex toys in the classifieds of various periodicals. Reputable vendors are discreet and will send your order in plain packaging; some even need a signature to confirm that it was delivered to the correct recipient.

You will learn how a sex toy will improve your enjoyment and encourage good sexual health by adding it into your sex life, whether it is for solo or couples play. Once you get going, you can find yourself having a drawer or cabinet full of stunning sex toys to satisfy every sex need and want.

How lubricant can transform your sex life: There appears to be a misconception that younger women do not require lubrication and if they do, they have a problem. However, lubricant may completely change your sex life. People use a number of strange chemicals as lubricants, but choosing the appropriate one may significantly alter the experience.

People may not desire sex for a variety of reasons, such as fatigue, discomfort, pain, lack of excitement, or just because it doesn't feel very enjoyable. People experiment with the most bizarre procedures and tools to enhance their sex lives, from purchasing the priciest, all-singing, all-dancing sex toy to swinging from the ceiling while wearing a Wonder Woman costume.

Most people associate the word "lubricant" with older women who experience vaginal dryness during the menopause (due to a decline in oestrogen), but sexual lubricants can be beneficial for men and women of any age.

It's important to dispel the misconception that lubricants are only required to "fix" sexual issues. Young or old, many women experience vaginal dryness at some point in their lives but are too self-conscious to talk about it or get help.

Sadly, there seems to be a false perception spread by social media and the general public that younger women do not require vaginal lubrication because they should always be moist and should seek medical attention if they are not.

Vaginal secretion levels vary among women and can be influenced by a variety of factors, including:

- Stress, anxiety, and relationship problems Hormonal changes brought on by contraception, pregnancy, breastfeeding, and menstruation
- Medical conditions like diabetes, chemotherapy side effects, a full hysterectomy, or immune disorders.
- Chemical goods such as washing powders, abrasive soaps, feminine sprays or douches, and perfumed toilet paper
- Drugs such as the contraceptive pill, anti-depressants, and allergy medications
- Lack of foreplay
- The fact that women require greater stimulation than males.

Generally speaking, women felt positively about lubricants, preferring that sex feel more moist than not, according to a 2013 research of 2,451 females between the ages of 18 and 68. Nine out of ten women said that applying lubricant made sex more enjoyable, pleasant, and overall better.

Additionally, it can make sex enjoyable for guys as well. The sensitive tissues of the vagina and penis are protected from harm or abrasion by having a well-lubricated penis, which also improves enjoyment. If the sexual encounter is enjoyable, it may also lengthen.

Erection and arousal issues are a problem for older men as well. The use of lubrication can heighten pleasure and lengthen erections because it requires longer genital arousal to achieve erections and be turned on. You can heighten arousal and increase pleasure by using lubricants during foreplay or when you are unable to engage in penetrative sex.

Which lubricant should I use?
I advise applying a lubricant while using sex toys, and I frequently hear about a wide range of unusual items, including butter, margarine, hand

cream, vegetable and massage oils, baby oil, petroleum jelly (Vaseline), and saliva.

Many consumers fail to take into account the potential ingredients in these products, some of which might irritate skin or create allergies or thrush. Many couples use saliva as lubrication, but it rapidly dries out and is more watery than slick.

You should think carefully about the lubricant you choose since some lubricants that tingle or are coloured might irritate or induce allergic responses in some people. Nothing is worse than a burning penis or vagina.

Water based lubricants:
These are the most adaptable lubricant kinds since they may be used with silicone sex objects and are safe for all sexual activities. These are the most widely used options because they are affordable, non-staining, and many can be consumed in small amounts during sex. They

can also be used safely with latex diaphragms and condoms.

Additionally, water-based lubricants have the advantage of being exceedingly simple to remove after usage, leaving your skin clean, velvety smooth, and residue-free. You may add a bit extra if they start to dry up or use water to revive them.

Oil-based lubricants:
Because they are thicker and more creamy in texture, oil-based lubricants stay longer during sex and provide a superb, long-lasting, silky smooth feeling. Although they are excellent for masturbating, you should be aware that they should not be used with latex contraception. During sexual activity, both water- and oil-based lubricants can be used.

Silicone-based lubricants:
They are fantastic for having fun in the water and are safe to use with latex condoms. They also last a very long time. However, because

they will harm the surface, they should not be used on silicone sex toys. Give Lube silicone-based lubricant is moisturizing, dermatologist-approved, and free of preservatives.

Petroleum-based lubricants:
It is advised to stay away from petroleum-based products since they are difficult to remove and may irritate the vagina by altering the pH, which can cause yeast infections. In addition, they damage latex and condoms.

Some lubricants come in tubes and applicators, making it simpler to administer the lubricant precisely where you want it to go. A little goes a long way. Finally, before putting it directly on the genitals, warm it up by squirting a tiny bit into your fingers.

Chapter 7

GENERAL TIPS

There are several things you can do to get your sex life back on track, regardless of how large or minor the issue is. Your general physical, mental, and emotional health are all closely related to your sexual well-being. You may get through difficult times by talking to your spouse, leading a healthy lifestyle, utilizing some of the many fantastic self-help resources available to you, and simply having fun.

Having a fulfilling sexual life:

So - The term has a wide range of emotional connotations. The emotions to sexual encounters range from love, pleasure, and compassion to desire, worry, and disappointment. Furthermore, many people will experience all of these feelings as well as a host of others during the course of a sexual life that lasts for several decades.

But what exactly is sex?

On a basic level, sex is merely another hormonally-driven biological process intended to ensure the survival of the species. Naturally, this limited perspective undervalues the complexity of the human sexual response. Your experiences and expectations, in addition to the biological factors at play, determine your sexuality. Your capacity to build and sustain a healthy sex life will largely depend on your perception of yourself as a sexual person, your ideas about what makes a good sexual connection, and your relationship with your partner.

Speaking to your partner:

Even in the best of circumstances, discussing sex may be challenging for many couples. Sexual issues may cause hurt, shame, guilt, and animosity, which can completely stop communication. Establishing a conversation is the first step to a healthier sex life as well as a tighter emotional link since effective communication is the foundation of a successful relationship. Here are some suggestions for handling this delicate topic.

- Choose a suitable moment to speak: Sexual talks may be divided into two categories: those that take place in the bedroom and those that take place outside of it. When you're in the middle of making love, it's absolutely OK to tell your partner what makes you feel good, but it's better to hold off on talking about more significant concerns like incompatible sexual desires or orgasm issues until you're in a more neutral environment.

- Avoid being critical: Instead of focusing on the cons, couch suggestions in positive terms like, "I really love it when you lightly touch my hair that way." Instead of seeing a sexual issue as an opportunity to place blame, approach it as a problem that has to be tackled jointly.

- Tell your spouse about physical changes you're experiencing, such as hot flashes that keep you up at night or dry vagina brought on by menopause. Knowing what's truly happening is vastly preferable than misinterpreting these bodily changes as loss of interest. Show your spouse how to arouse you instead of letting her think she isn't attractive enough to do so any longer if you're a male and you no longer get an erection only from the notion of sex.

- Be truthful: By pretending to have an orgasm, you may believe you are protecting your partner's feelings, but in reality, you are only beginning to tread dangerous ground. As difficult as it is to discuss any sexual issue, the challenge multiplies when the problem is buried behind years of deceit, grief, and hatred.

- Don't equate love with sexual performance: Create a loving and tender atmosphere by frequently touching and kissing. Don't put the blame for your inability to have sex on your spouse or yourself. Instead, put your attention on preserving the emotional and physical intimacy in your union. What will happen once one spouse passes away is another potentially delicate topic that is worthwhile of discussion for older couples. The surviving spouse in a good sex-filled relationship will probably wish to find a new companion. The procedure will likely be easier on the surviving spouse afterwards if you express your openness to that idea while you are both still living.

- Using self-help techniques: Treating sexual issues is now simpler than ever. If you need them, cutting-edge drugs and qualified sex therapists are available. However, by making a few changes to your lovemaking technique, you might be able to address minor sexual problems.

- Learn more: There are a ton of excellent self-help resources available for all kinds of sexual issues. You and your spouse can utilize a few resources you find while browsing the Internet or your neighborhood bookshop to learn more about the issue. You and your companion can highlight portions that you find particularly compelling and display them to each other if speaking directly is too tough.

- Internet use and privacy issues: The Internet is a great resource for finding all kinds of information, including books and other goods (such sex devices that can improve your sex life). Although it may seem obvious, never conduct such searches on a work computer to avoid embarrassing your employer, who is probably able to track your search history. People who are uncomfortable about ordering sex-related information or items online using their home computers and credit cards may be able to locate a local store (particularly in big cities) and pay with cash.

- Allow yourself some time because sexual arousal decreases with age: In order to increase your chances of success, you and your partner should look for a place for sex that is peaceful, relaxing, and free from distractions. Additionally, be aware that it will take you longer to become aroused and have orgasm due to the physical changes to your body. When you give it some thought, having more sex isn't always a negative thing; incorporating these bodily requirements into your romantic routine might lead to new types of sexual experiences.

- Use lubrication: As was mentioned in the previous chapter, lubricating liquids and gels may frequently be used to treat the dryness of the vagina that appears during perimenopause. Use these freely to prevent uncomfortable sex, an issue that can develop into a waning libido and escalating marital conflicts. Talk to your doctor about additional choices if lubricants stop working.

- Maintain physical affection: Kissing and cuddling are crucial for preserving an emotional and physical link, even when you're exhausted, anxious, or irritated about the issue.

- Practice touching: You may re-establish physical closeness without feeling pressed by using the sensate concentration techniques used by sex therapists. These exercises may be found in a variety of self-help books and instructional DVDs. Additionally, you might want to request that your spouse touch you in the manner in which he or she like to be touched. This can help you determine the appropriate level of pressure to apply, from light to hard.

- Try new positions: As earlier discussed in chapter 4, experimenting with different sexual positions not only makes romantic relationships more interesting, but it may also assist in resolving issues. For instance, when a guy enters his partner from behind, the greater stimulation to the G-spot that results might assist the woman in reaching orgasm.

- The G-spot, also known as the Grafenberg spot after the gynecologist who originally discovered it, is a mound of extraordinarily sensitive tissue that may be found immediately inside the vagina's opening in the roof of the vagina. Effective G-spot stimulation can result in powerful orgasms. The G-spot is not routinely activated for the majority of women during vaginal sex due to its challenging location and the fact that it is best stimulated manually. Research has shown that a different kind of tissue does exist in this area, despite some skeptics' doubts to the contrary.

- To find your G-spot, you must be sexually aroused: If you're crouching or sitting down, try beckoning your finger along the roof of your vagina. If not, ask your partner to massage the top of your vagina until they feel a particularly sensitive place. Some women are more sensitive and can easily find the spot, but for some it's challenging.

- You shouldn't be concerned if you have trouble finding it. Many women believe that entering from behind will more readily trigger the G-spot during sex. Playing with the G-spot might improve romantic interactions for couples who have erection issues. An extremely powerful orgasm can be produced in a woman by oral stimulation of the clitoris and manual stimulation of the G-spot.

- Write down your fantasies to explore potential actions that you believe would turn you or your lover on. Consider an event or a movie that stirred your emotions, then share that memory with your partner. For those who have little desire, this is especially beneficial.

- Perform Kegel exercises: By strengthening the pelvic floor muscles, both men and women can increase their sexual fitness. To do these exercises, tense the same muscle that you would if you were attempting to halt the flow of pee. Release after holding the contraction for two to three seconds. Ten times in total. Aim to perform five sets each day. You can perform these exercises anywhere, whether you're driving, working at your desk, or waiting in a checkout line. Vaginal weights can be used by women at home to increase muscle resistance. Find out where to get them and how to use them by speaking with your doctor or a sex therapist.

- Try to unwind: Before engaging in sexual activity, engage in something calming together, like playing a game or going out to a nice dinner. Alternately, experiment with relaxing methods like yoga or deep breathing exercises.

- Use a vibrator to express your preferences to your spouse. A vibrator may teach you about your own sexual reaction.

- If none of your efforts seem to be working, don't lose hope. Your doctor may be able to identify the root of your sexual issue and suggest effective treatments. He or she can also connect you with a sex therapist who can assist you in examining any problems that might be getting in the way of having satisfying sexual relations.

- Keeping one's health: Your general physical, mental, and emotional health are all closely related to your sexual well-being. Therefore, the same healthy behaviors that you use to maintain the health of your body may also improve your sexual life.

- Exercise, exercise, exercise: Among the healthy habits that might enhance your sexual performance, physical activity comes top. Exercise that builds heart and blood vessel strength, which is essential for physical arousal, is aerobic exercise. And exercise has a ton of additional health advantages, like preventing heart disease, osteoporosis, and some types of cancer, as well as elevating your mood and promoting better sleep. Don't forget to incorporate strength training as well.

- Avoid smoking: Smoking increases the risk of peripheral vascular disease, which affects the tissues of the penis, clitoris, and vagina. Additionally, smokers typically experience menopause two years earlier than non-smokers do. Try nicotine gum or patches to help you stop smoking, or talk to your doctor about bupropion (Zyban) or varenicline (Chantix).

- Drink less alcohol: Some erectile dysfunctional men discover that a single drink can help them unwind, but binge drinking can exacerbate the condition. Because it dulls the central nervous system, alcohol can prevent sexual responses. Large amounts of alcohol consumed over an extended period of time can harm the liver, increasing the synthesis of estrogen in males. Alcohol might worsen menopausal symptoms in women by causing hot flashes and disrupting sleep.

- Eating poorly causes high blood cholesterol and obesity, both of which are significant risk factors for cardiovascular disease. Additionally, being overweight might encourage sluggishness and a negative self-image. Losing those excess pounds frequently has the added benefit of enhancing libido.

- Use it or lose it: The flexibility of the vaginal walls decreases when estrogen levels fall after menopause. Through sexual intercourse, you can halt or even reverse this process. Masturbation is equally as effective if having sex is not an option, albeit for women, it works best if you use a vibrator or dildo (an instrument that resembles a penis to help expand the vagina). Long stretches without an erection in males can deprive the penis of some of the oxygen-rich blood it need to keep healthy sexual function. As a result, muscle cells start to resemble scar tissue, which prevents the penis from expanding when blood flow is increased.

- Restoring the joy of sex: Even in the ideal relationship, sex may get stale after a while. You can reignite the flame with a little bit of creative thinking.

- Be daring: If you've never had sex on the living room floor or in a remote area of the woods, this could be the perfect opportunity. or look into erotic literature and cinema. You could get horny even simply from the naughty vibe you get from renting an X-rated movie.

- Be sensual: Set up a romantic setting that satisfies all five of your senses. Focus on the sensation of silk on your skin, the rhythm of jazz music, the floral fragrance filling the space, the mellow glow of candlelight, and the flavor of ripe, luscious fruit. When making love to your partner, make use of this increased sensual awareness.

- Be playful and tuck love notes into your partner's pocket for later discovery. Take a bubble bath together; the snug, warm sensation you experience after getting out the tub may be a terrific prelude to sex. Tickle. Laugh!

- Be innovative: Variate your scripts and broaden your sexual repertoire. If you typically make love on Saturday night, for instance, pick Sunday morning instead. Try out different roles and pursuits. If you've never used sex toys or sexy lingerie, give them a try.

- Consider reading poems to one another while seated next to a tree on a hillside. When there is no special occasion, surprise each other with flowers. Plan a day where you do nothing but talk and cuddle in bed. Your perspective on sexuality is the most crucial tool you possess. With the right knowledge and a positive attitude, you should be able to sustain a fulfilling sexual life for many years to come.

Chapter 8

SEXUAL SELF ESTEEM
(Overcoming Shyness)

Sexual self-esteem is the general assessment of one's own value that is known as self-esteem. It covers how individuals feel about their emotions, self-beliefs, and how those things show themselves in their behaviors. It has been determined that self-esteem is essential—even indispensable—to regular and balanced self-development. What connection does this have to sexuality? This almost always manifests itself sexually in the same way. Our attitudes, feelings, and actions may resemble inquiries like these:

Am I overweight?
Do I look decent?
Do I make my sweetheart happy?
Are they enjoying themselves?
Do my fantasies seem too odd?
Why do I feel so guilty and ashamed?
Am I unfaithful?

Some of these sexual self-esteem issues might cause us to have irrational expectations about how we view our bodies, our relationships, and sex in general. It is difficult to appreciate the intimacy and thrill that come with healthy sexual encounters if they are a reflection of poor self-esteem. A person needs analyze a few personal ideas (typically done in sex therapy) in order to develop a healthy and vigorous sexual self-esteem, such as:

How your physical and emotional well-being affect your capacity to prefer engaging in sex to performing it. Sex may be entertaining, occasionally embarrassing, private, passionate, and a variety of other things. The success of your performance will depend far more on the experience of these adjectives. When you concentrate on your performance, such as your form, endurance, how loud you scream or don't scream, comparisons to porn stars, etc., you'll be less able to truly appreciate the moment you're supposed to be experiencing.

an emphasis on enjoying your body for the pleasure it gives you and your partner rather than just its appearance. Do you actually believe that your significant other is concerned about the extra dimple on your butt cheek or whether the lighting makes your breasts appear uneven? It's unlikely that this is where your lover is now concentrating their attention. They are there because they like your body; you need to feel the same way.

Make it a practice to appreciate your physical and emotional well-being. Does this imply that you should enhance your habit of masturbating? No, but it does imply that you should value yourself more. A higher sense of sexual self-worth is being comfortable in your own skin, both inside and outside of clothing, loving your perfection and imperfections, and realizing that your individual needs necessitate a special sexual creation. Finding the aspects of your body that you value and like will help you achieve this. Spend some time gazing at your body in the mirror.

It's absurd to ask yourself things like, "Am I fat?" or "Do I look good?" Your partner is making an effort to get close to you because they obviously think you look good. People are typically not motivated to engage in sexual activity with someone they are not attracted to. So, change these ideas to "I look beautiful, my body looks wonderful, and I am hot" and let your mind and body have a fantastic time. Being truthful with your spouse is one method to facilitate this. Tell them if they are touching you in a way that makes you uncomfortable or distracts you from the present. They might not be aware of it, and they won't find out unless you tell them. By highlighting your good qualities, reclaim control over how you feel about your body. We've all got them.

Various more questions, such "Do I fulfill my lover?" and "Are they enjoying themselves?" reduce sexual self-esteem since your partner will enjoy themselves if you enjoy yourself. The capacity to abandon caution and fully immerse oneself in the encounter is a crucial component of the sexual experience. People find that personal freedom and confidence to be seductive, alluring, and rewarding.

In terms of feelings like shame and guilt related to past sexual experiences or fantasies, the moment is not the right place to feel them. Even though it's understandable that they might affect one's sexual self-esteem, if it really bothers you, try to deal with it before engaging in sexual activity. In order to better understand the emotional pattern you go through, what causes these emotions, and potential solutions, you might want to journal about your past if it still haunts you.

Therefore, Sex Therapy in Philadelphia has established several tried-and-true methods to raise good ideas, pleasant emotions, and positive actions in order to boost your sexual self-esteem:

A excellent notion to have is that I make a decent lover. Whatever your speciality, whether it be a wonderful kiss, a decent massage, a soft touch, or a fantastic lick, it helps to identify you as a lover. Celebrate your expertise and move forward.

It makes me feel good to believe in a sexual god or goddess. Although it seems cliche, praising oneself with phrases like "I am good enough and people like me" actually works. Understanding that you are not less than anybody is essential to developing a healthy and happy sexual self-esteem. Feeling like a sexual god or goddess may help you feel seductive, seductive, and intriguing. Who could not enjoy that?

A good attitude to display is "I'm going to live in this moment." Living in the present is essential for developing a healthy sexual self-esteem. Live in the now rather than trying to forecast the future or concentrate on the past.

A pleasant emotion is when I feel nice. Despite sounding unimportant, it is crucial for fostering strong sexual self-esteem. When you are about to have or are experiencing a sexual encounter, feeling good might help you relax and become more aware of your body's sensations and reactions.

One of the most crucial ideas to have is that "my body is my temple" and that "I am in command of this experience." Whatever your sexual gratification, it's crucial to control the experience. This does not imply that you must actually initiate any sexual activity, but rather that you are in charge of deciding what is and is not acceptable depending on your comfort levels.

Recognize that this is not a comprehensive list of constructive attitudes, sensations, or actions. You are developing YOUR sexual self-esteem, so use this as a beginning point or a reference when creating your own list. Just keep in mind that you are deserving of wonderful sex, deserving of feeling good, and deserving of experiencing the experience repeatedly as you build your sexual self-esteem.

Chapter 9

SEX TABOOS

12 Poor Practices That Are Ruining Your Sexual Life

Do you watch Netflix more often than your partner? That is a difficulty.

Sex should undoubtedly be more than simply another task to complete. But with the craziness of work, raising children, and daily life, you occasionally need to come up with a strategy to, well, make it happen. Furthermore, it's simple to allow the minor things to get in the way. Hey, we all commit a few of them.

1. Cuddling in bed with your iPad:
Yes, it might be challenging to stop using Pinterest or to resist binge-watching the newest Orange Is the New Black season. But time, passion, and emotional energy can be lost to technology. Many women claim they have no time for sex, but Andrea Syrtash, a relationship

specialist and the author of Cheat on Your Husband, notes that many admit to checking Facebook an hour before bed (With Your Husband). Additionally, sending that final email before turning down the lights ensures that you are concentrating on your work and not on getting into bed with your spouse. Dr. Jane Greer, a marital and sex therapist in New York, argues that this means that emotionally, you are elsewhere. (Having a TV in the bedroom is also ineffective: Couples only have sex half as often, according to a recent research!) To reduce distractions, both experts advise turning off your electronics an hour before bed.

2. Eating excessively or too late:

According to Dr. Rachel A. Sussman, LCSW, stress and hectic schedules both contribute to late meals, midnight snacking, and overeating. "Those behaviors may make us drained, stuffed, and self-conscious." What occurs when we don't feel good about ourselves, do you know? a great deal of nothing. she gave? Consider sex as your dessert, Sussman exhorts. There is a very strong probability that you will have more energy and desire to have sex later that evening if you eat less. (Also, you can always follow with something sweet.)

3. Pouring another glass of wine:

Drinking alcohol is another cunning offender that can be snuffing out your enthusiasm. According to Sussman, "people frequently drink to manage stress, but it might backfire, leaving them fatigued or grumpy." Why? as alcohol has a depressive effect. However, not all alcoholic beverages are unhealthy; just be mindful of your intake. Sussman continues, "A little bit can excite you on, but too much can definitely destroy a sex drive and make it hard to climax.

4. Sleeping in the bed with the dog or cat:

We understand it. The puppy-dog eyes are difficult to avoid. However, Virginia Sadock, M.D., Director of the Program in Human Sexuality at NYU Langone Medical Center, advises against bringing dogs into the bedroom. In fact, your dog could gain from giving you some breathing room. Pets, like kids, don't appreciate being left out, but Sadock observes that they dislike parental conflict even less. And since having sex helps reduce stress, shut the door for the evening.

5. Being a one-trick pony:

Its true that monogamy might get boring after a while. Routines are simple to get into, especially if you find one that "works," but restraining yourself from repeating the same moves can help keep you interested in playing again. Sussman advises doing some reading, experimenting with different body postures, or coming up with original techniques to entice your partner: "It doesn't need to be difficult. As simple as flirting can do it."

6. Always traveling with the kids:

If you're always traveling with children, Disney World will typically be preferred over Aruba. However, a February 2013 research commissioned by the U.S. Travel Association found that couples who travel together at least once a year had more contented sexual lives. More closeness may be sparked by just one weekend get-away than by giving tiny presents. So instead of giving gifts of love, save your money and spend it on a vacation.

7. Putting on your cozy pajamas:

That baggy shirt or prairie-chic plaid dress are probably not helping either of you feel particularly motivated. Syrtash notes that wearing gorgeous underwear might make sexual activity feel more seductive. "If you often wear granny pants to bed, try switching it up with sensuous materials that feel wonderful on your skin. You'll feel sensuous, and he'll think it's sexy." Therefore, everyone benefits.

8. Self-criticism destroys libido:

Everyone undoubtedly has a "problem region" on their body that they don't like. Not to mention that doing it in front of your lover is not the sexiest thing to do. According to clinical psychologist and AASECT Certified Sex Therapist Dr. Shannon Chavez, "giving yourself negative messages about your body every time you look in the mirror can lower your mood, well-being, and deplete your energy." Instead, be positive about your appearance and get to work. You'll feel better afterward, we guarantee.

9. Skipping the gym:

Being confident does not entail letting everything go: According to Sadock, "moderate exercise helps you build up stamina, it gives you energy, and it is also a fantastic method to release anxiety." The more energy you have left over to feel aroused about sex, the less energy you are using on feeling nervous. An added bonus: A University of Florida study found that post-workout sex can be fantastic. Why? Even if you haven't dropped any weight, you end up feeling more confident and liberated. According to science.

10. Not Scheduling your "special time":

Although it may not sound romantic, organizing your bedtime antics improves them, frequently by removing guilt. "It's easy to feel like you always have something more important to be doing than having sex if you're a really busy person, especially a stay-at-home mom or a working mom," Sussman claims, adding that she advises arranging couples' time at least once a week.

11. Passing up those small opportunities to connect:

You may also revive your libido outside of the bedroom. According to Sadock, lunch dates are particularly helpful for helping couples reconnect on a deeper level. "Twenty minutes of chatting — when you're not washing the dishes, folding clothes, or watching TV — helps you reconnect with your spouse on a deeper level," she says. Because it's a respite during the day and you're not as worn out as you are at night, it is inherently unique.

12. Don't wait for the ideal time:

Act now. Seriously. The decline in estrogen levels that occurs in women as they age, as well as after giving birth, can cause dryness in the vagina and decreased desire. However, starting to kiss and fondle while being out of the mood might really turn you on. You may thank us later if you try it.

Chapter 10

SAFETY

Top Ten Tips for Safer Sex

How can we explore our sexuality, have fun with it, and stay healthy at the same time? The majority of us have, at some time, forgotten to apply protection even though the majority of us are aware of the simple solutions. Use the advice provided here to keep yourself safe at all times.

1. BYOC: Bring your own condom; don't rely on your companion to provide lubricant or condoms. Always have some on hand, and before using, make sure to check the expiration dates.

2. Have safer-sex role-playing chats with friends: You may become more confident and aggressive when the time comes to speak about it in person by rehearsing what to say and coming up with coping mechanisms for dealing with challenging reactions. The ideal

suggestions and counsel can come from those who have had similar situations and who actually comprehend your worries.

3. Establish fundamental restrictions and boundaries in advance of safer sex: You may be reminded that they are crucial and non-negotiable by writing them down.

4. Avoid being so inebriated or euphoric that you risk making bad decisions.

5. Make safer sex an integral part of sex rather than a separate activity: Use condoms, either male or female, together, as an example.

6. Take your time with lower- or no-risk activities first, which helps foster dialogue and trust. Then go on to higher-risk activities (and also feel really good).

7. Seek the assistance of a therapist, counselor, or support group to aid you in your recovery and to help you choose partners and sexual

environments that make you feel at ease if you have a history of sexual or other abuse and believe that this interferes with your capacity to be safe.

8. Pick partners who don't place the onus of safer sex solely on you: Consider working with partners who are open to discussing safety.

9. Strive to be more comfortable discussing sex and sexual health with friends and lovers. When you don't feel ashamed, it's simpler to be safe.

10. If you have trouble with this, don't feel awful about yourself: Many of us were taught that decent females don't talk about sex or that it's not romantic to do so. However, we are able to do so, and with experience, it becomes simpler.